The Practical Caregiver's Guide to Rock Star Caregiving: How to Help Someone Who Is Seriously Ill

SARA M. BARTON

Copyright © 2018 Sara M. Barton

All rights reserved.

ISBN: 198667777X
ISBN-13: 978-1986677776

DEDICATION

For all of my cancer friends, who have taught me that real support is all about being there every step of the way. Never stop believing that life can be better. When you keep hope alive, you seek the opportunities that will nurture your soul.

And never forget that tomorrow is promised to no one. We have this moment in time. It is up to us to live it well.

CONTENTS

Introduction	1
Chapter One -- Why Join the Band?	3
Chapter Two -- Think Like a Band Manager	5
Chapter Three -- Know Your Players	10
Chapter Four -- Learning to Negotiate and Placate	13
Chapter Five -- Our Signature Songs Define Us	16
Chapter Six -- I Wasn't Prepared for This Gig	20
Chapter Seven -- What Happens Offstage?	24
Chapter Eight -- Life in a Fish Bowl	28
Chapter Nine -- Groupies, Sickies, and Needies	31
Chapter Ten -- It's Not All about You and Yet It Is	35
Chapter Eleven -- Can You Die from Stage Fright?	39
Chapter Twelve-- How Did We Fall into This Hole?	42
Chapter Thirteen -- I Used to Be Somebody	45
Chapter Fourteen -- Celebrity Sightings and Other Freak Outs	48
Chapter Fifteen -- Championing a Cause Only Works If It Fixes a Problem	52

Chapter Sixteen -- What a Long, Strange Trip It's Been   57

Author Information   60

INTRODUCTION

What do rock stars and seriously ill people have in common? They need good managers to help them survive their sometimes chaotic lives.

To be a rock star, you have to know something about music. To be a caregiver, you have to know something about care. To be a rock star caregiver, you have to go deep into the soul and bring out the music there, by making life as copacetic as possible for someone with serious health needs.

Every rock star has to do two things on a regular basis. You have to practice your music and you have to perform it. The more you practice, the better you perform. The more you perform, the better the music sounds.

Every rock star caregiver goes above and beyond all that. You have to practice your caregiving skills and you have to improve on them, especially as your loved one struggles with escalating challenges. The more you practice, the better your care. The more you care, the better the care you provide.

If you're caring for someone debilitated by a serious illness, you understand how complicated it is for your loved one to keep going on a daily basis. The challenges are often enormous and difficult; they use up a lot of precious energy. Your loved one probably goes back and forth to doctor's offices, treatments, and even to the ER when unexpected problems crop up.

No doubt your loved one has an entourage, just like a real rock star. There are peeps to do this and peeps to do that. But you, as the main caregiver, are the go-to person. The days of going solo are over for someone who is seriously ill. Without you, there is no music. You may not be the star of the show, friend, but you are an important part of keeping the music alive.

CHAPTER ONE -- WHY JOIN THE BAND?

Sure, you've got a stellar career (or retirement) of your own. You have an active schedule. You're achieving your goals. Life is good. Why would you change any of that to take care of a loved one with a serious illness?

Why not just hire someone to do it? That way, you don't have to worry about a thing. Just farm the job out and get on with your own life. But is that the best option?

Consider this. You're talking about someone who's also had an impressive life, wonderful achievements, stellar talents, and amazing skills. And then suddenly all of that is upended in an ugly heap. Maybe it's your spouse who has cancer. Maybe it's your parent with heart disease. Maybe it's your best friend with Parkinson's...or your cousin with MS...or your sibling with any of a number of diseases or illnesses. Why, oh why, would you voluntarily sacrifice your own life to take care of someone you love?

There's the key word -- love. Love makes the world go round. It makes us do things we never thought possible, good and bad. It drives us to new heights and sinks us to new lows. Above all, it motivates us to do for others. If we're smart, we understand what our lives would be like without it.

When rock stars show up on stage and perform flawlessly, it's easy to think that talent is the only requirement that makes the magic. But behind every rock star, there are a number of people hard at work, making it possible for that show to go on. The same is true for seriously ill patients.

The logistics of managing a band can be complicated. If you're in a garage band, just playing local gigs on weekends, your commitment of time, money, and energy is likely to be minimal. But if you're part of a successful musical group that tours nationally or internationally, your responsibilities increase considerably.

The same can be said for helping a loved one manage an illness. If your loved one doesn't have many symptoms or challenges, you're not going to be all that involved with the care your loved one receives. But if he or she is seriously ill, you may find yourself constantly juggling crises and issues.

CHAPTER TWO -- THINK LIKE A BAND MANAGER

A band manager usually wears several hats for the band. It's all about logistics. You make sure the bills get paid on time and the travel arrangements get booked. You hire roadies to do the heavy lifting, moving equipment from stage to stage. There are sound checks and rehearsals to get through. The local media might want interviews, so the publicist needs to schedule access to the members. You worry about food for the band members and the roadies. The bigger the rock star, the bigger the entourage.

Fans want the chance to see the rock star perform in person. The band manager has to oversee the bookings. There's nothing worse than putting the band into the wrong venue. If you book a concert hall that's too big, there will be many empty seats and little profit. That can really kill the vibe. Pick a club that's too small and you won't have enough seats for attendees. You will, however, have disgruntled fans that you will need to mollify.

In caregiving, it's important to understand that medical appointments are a huge part of any seriously ill patient's life, and booking them effectively can be challenging.

Some appointments are easy to handle. If the doctor is on schedule and there are no complications, your loved one will breeze through it.

Some appointments are harder. If the doctor is running late because of a previous emergency, your loved one may have to wait. What if it will be an hour or more? Is it feasible to stay or should the appointment be rebooked? That will depend on the patient's energy level, the reason for seeing the doctor, and the next available appointment.

Some doctors become redundant when the challenges of managing the serious illness intensify. If your dad routinely sees his dermatologist for minor skin cancers, it might not be necessary to continue with that now that he's been diagnosed with prostate cancer. The oncologist who is treating him at the cancer center can take over the responsibility.

Then again, if your loved one's health is complicated by a serious illness, you might just find that there are *more* medical professionals called in to manage all the symptoms and complications that arise. You might find yourself thrust into the role of coordinator, insuring that all of the doctors are informed of the patient's situation in a crisis. If your dad has a vascular scan, it's important that the primary care physician gets a copy of the results. But so, too, should his cardiologist, because any problems could also impact his heart. If your mom is being treated for pneumonia by the primary care physician, the oncologist needs to know, because it could affect her regular chemotherapy schedule. She might need to postpone treatments. And that blood clot your husband developed in his lung will be of interest not only to his vascular surgeon, but also to his pulmonologist. Which doctor should treat it?

The treatments have to get booked properly. It sounds easy enough, but do you know what time of day your loved one has the most energy? Or when your loved one needs to crash for a nap? Or when medications need to be taken? If you want your loved one to make it through that treatment, you'll need to make sure you time the appointments appropriately.

But booking the appointment isn't all you have to do. Is a referral required by the insurance company for certain treatments or to see certain doctors? Imagine taking your loved one to the hospital for what appears to be a routine treatment, only to find that it hasn't yet been approved by the insurance company. Not only is your loved one stressed by the news, he or she has wasted valuable energy preparing for something that's not going to happen. You have to make sure you know whether there is a referral in place before you go. In some cases, the scheduler will let you know it hasn't come through yet, but this isn't always the case. It never hurts to call ahead and make sure.

But what if the referral hasn't come through and the physician's office suggests your loved one signs a waiver in the hope that the insurance company will provide one *after* the treatment proceeds? Know this. If the insurance company does not feel the treatment is essential, your loved one will be stuck with the payment for the entire treatment.

What if the insurance company and the hospital are in the middle of contract negotiations and they fail to come to an agreement by the deadline? Did you know that your loved one's physicians might suddenly be booted out of the network by the insurer? If that is the case, continuing treatment with those physicians will create enormous financial headaches. Will your loved one have to switch doctors to be treated?

Do you know which of your loved one's physicians handle which conditions? That may sound like a silly thing to ask, but seriously ill patients often wind up being treated by several overlapping specialists for multiple conditions. If there are heart problems, the cardiologist might be the go-to doc. But if it's a vascular issue, it could be the vascular surgeon who is called in. If that chemo is creating physical complications, you might need to contact the oncologist. But what if your loved one is short of breath or in pain because of a blood clot? You bounce back to the cardiologist and the vascular surgeon. It can be nerve-racking, when things are going badly, to try to figure out which doctor to call.

Your loved one is probably on a number of medications that have serious side effects. Very often, doctors will prescribe them anyway, because the illness is so debilitating. When complications arise, it can be very difficult to identify the medication that is creating the dangerous complication or side effect. This is why it's so important to know the name and dosage of every medication dispensed at home *and* dispensed in a medical setting. Sometimes information slips through the cracks. Someone fails to read a medical chart. The more you understand about each treatment and the complications that might arise, the better you will perform during a crisis.

Each doctor on your loved one's medical team should receive test results that are relevant to his or her specialty. It can save a lot of time, money, and your loved one's energy in the long run, especially if the doctors can share test results and avoid duplicating scans, x-rays, and other diagnostic procedures. Being on top of the information solidifies your reputation as the go-to person.

CHAPTER THREE -- KNOW YOUR PLAYERS

A successful band manager needs to know some specifics about the music business. How dedicated are the fans? Are they willing to travel to shows or do they prefer to only venture out locally? Do they spend money for tickets or will they only opt for the inexpensive seats in the nosebleed section? Do they like outdoor or indoor concerts? The tour has to make a profit, so the band manager has to focus on the financial bottom line, making sure that the bookings will produce the desired result -- improving the rock star's fan base, enhancing the public image, and most of all, providing a good entertainment experience for everyone involved.

A successful rock star caregiver also needs to appreciate the logistics of being seriously ill. Not every physician is a good fit for every patient. Some physicians are notorious for deliberately overbooking; they run late on a regular basis and that can waste your loved one's precious time and energy. Once in the exam room, the physician may hurry through the process, leaving your loved one feeling like a statistic, instead of a valued patient.

Time constraints can also be a factor. The physician's office might be so far away, it takes up too much time to go back and forth. What if there is an emergency? Will your loved one have the stamina to travel? When it comes to serious illness, sometimes it's important to find the best of the specialists available in your local area to treat your loved one.

Good health care isn't something that *happens* to patients. Doctors don't get to dictate what treatments patients will undergo. Patients *choose* what they are willing to endure, especially when they are seriously ill. It's a partnership between patient and provider. There can be personality conflicts with some doctors. How should these be handled? If the physician has a strong opinion as to how your loved one's illness should be managed and the patient balks, what can you do? A patient has to feel invested in the treatment plan and the outcome. Every decision about what kind of care is received has to be agreed upon by the patient. If time, money, and energy are directed at survival, but the patient feels there is no quality of life, what good does it do your loved one? Your rock star patient has to believe that all of the struggling is worth the result.

Being seriously ill can be very costly and disrupt the flow of money coming in and going out of the household. If you and your loved one have to cut back on your hours or take unpaid leaves from work, it's going to affect your incomes. The bills and the co-pays for treatments can quickly add up. Most prescribed medications are covered by insurance, often with reasonable co-pays, but a lot of physicians now direct patients to take over-the-counter medications, and those are usually out-of-pocket expenses. With serious illness, there is often no time table for when a loved one is going to be better, or no guarantee that will happen. No one wants to feel like a burden to family, and yet, when the financial bottom line is hit, it can seriously stress the patient, the caregiver, and the family. You will have to plan ahead for those contingencies.

CHAPTER FOUR -- LEARNING TO NEGOTIATE AND PLACATE

A successful band manager is usually a good negotiator, able to please the rock star and make sure the magic happens by working behind the scenes, smoothing ruffled feathers and greasing the wheels. The same is true for successful caregivers. Being seriously ill takes so much energy, it's often difficult for a patient to stay involved in activities. Without real quality of life, your loved one is left to sing that old Rolling Stones' hit, *Can't Get No Satisfaction.*

One way to avoid that situation is to eliminate or minimize unnecessary strife and stress for your loved one as much as possible. As good rock star caregivers, we sometimes have to put ourselves between a rock and a hard place to spare our loved ones from worry and anxiety.

Home should be a sanctuary, a healing environment that is warm, comforting, and above all else, accessible. Even if we hire home health aides, companions, nurses, and therapists come to the home, even if other relatives and friends volunteer to take our loved one for treatments and appointments, we are the hands-on "go-to person" for the seriously ill patient, We keep up with what is going on and we field issues as quickly as we can, so that problems don't fester.

Just like a band manager is on top of the day-to-day issues for the rock star, a rock star caregiver should want to make sure that everything is going smoothly for the patient. Those unexpected glitches can create problems. Bills have to get paid on time. If your loved one chooses to keep this responsibility and has the stamina to successfully complete the task, it's fine. But what if he or she just can't handle that responsibility any more? What if chemotherapy muddles the mind and creates confusion? You will either have to take it on yourself or you will have to delegate it to someone who is trustworthy and capable to deal with the finances. Delegating tasks is something a good rock star caregiver has to do on a regular basis.

Yes, there will be crises during your stint as a rock star caregiver. It is part and parcel of caring for someone who is seriously ill. You will often have to navigate some very tenuous situations and protect your loved one from unintentional harm, misinformation, and wrong diagnoses. Careful observations, clear thinking, and a calm demeanor are tools that help rock star caregivers keep a loved one safer under challenging circumstances.

Is your loved one satisfied with how things are going? Making peace with a serious illness can sometimes seem like an impossible task. Patients are often frustrated when their bodies don't function well. Many of them are "sick of being sick". How can you comfort someone who feels dreadful most of the time? It's usually an ever-evolving situation that requires you and your loved one to be flexible and creative. As much as you loved one hates what this illness has done to the body, it's even tougher on the psyche. Salve for the soul is as essential as salve for the physical wounds.

CHAPTER FIVE -- OUR SIGNATURE SONGS DEFINE US

When we see a rock star in concert, we want to be dazzled. How would we react if Ed Sheeran insisted on performing the mundane *Twinkle, Twinkle, Little Star* all the time, rather than the outstanding *All of the Stars*? He wouldn't be much of a rock star, would he?

As rock star caregivers, should we ask our loved ones to waste their time and energy on doing mundane tasks that don't really matter, or should we encourage them to go after their goals? Adaptability and accessibility are all about empowerment. When we eliminate any obstacles that tax our loved ones, it frees them to do what's important to them.

How do we make that happen? We tweak the home care environment to ease the burden for someone with limited mobility or energy.

THE PRACTICAL CAREGIVER'S GUIDE TO ROCK STAR CAREGIVING

Consider what happens when band managers book accommodations for rock stars. They don't settle for just any old hotel room or suite. They want the right mix of pampering and comfort. Is that accommodation too close to the pool? If so, the rock star might hear kids screaming endlessly while trying to sleep after the previous night's performance. Where is the elevator located? If it's too close, that rock star will be disturbed by the constant comings and goings of other guests and hotel staff. If it's too far, that rock star could get ambushed by overly enthusiastic groupies and fans on the long walk back to the room. Will the ice machine create a ruckus every time those cubes are dumped? Will the door on the fire door slam while the rock star is hoping for quiet time? A good band manager tries to err on the side of caution by knowing what the rock star needs and what the hotel offers.

Good rock star caregivers do the same for seriously ill patients, finding ways to pamper and comfort, as a way of keeping them on an even keel during times of stress. No two patients have the same requirements. You might also find that your loved one's needs shift as the health challenges wax and wane. What works at this moment in time might not work later on.

Patients who have trouble sleeping or who need extra rest usually need a quiet environment. They can't tolerate the constant disruptions of their sleep cycles. Other patients need socialization, not isolation, and are willing to tolerate more noise in exchange for being around other people. How do you know what your loved one really needs? Ask.

Rock stars on tour expect to be pampered during their hotel stays. Luxurious appointments, such as elegant bedding and plush mattresses, Jacuzzi tubs, and private balconies, are just some of the perks of bedding down in luxe digs. An attentive concierge can also arrange for a gourmet meal, a soothing massage, or an icy mojito.

Seriously ill patients often spend so much time at medical appointments or treatments, the time they spend recovering matters. Little things mean a lot. Comfort is one key to healing. Is your loved one prone to chills? It's important to have a blanket handy to provide warmth. Is your loved one hydrating adequately throughout the day? Putting a carafe of water and a glass on the bedside table helps. Is your loved one struggling to maintain his or her weight? Putting snacks within reach can encourage your loved one to nibble throughout the day.

If your loved one has physical limitations, you can find practical ways to make home more user-friendly. Adapt the environment by renting a stair lift, putting in a temporary ramp, or even modifying the bathroom. Rearrange the furniture in the main care room to make it more functional. Put what is needed within reach of the bed or arm chair if you want to empower your loved one. Make sure there is adequate and accessible storage close by, just for good measure.

If stair-climbing has become an impossible task and a stair lift is not feasible, why not move the sleeping quarters downstairs? And if your loved one can't walk down a long hallway easily, relocate the main care room to a room closer to a bathroom.

Adjustable beds that can be raised and lowered are a good choice for some patients. These can be found in furniture stores. In some cases, hospital beds might be the better choice, because they have railings that will prevent a loved one from falling out of bed. Check with your loved one's insurance company to see if it's covered.

Other patients prefer to keep their own beds, for comfort or sentimental reasons. These can still be adapted with installed rails.

Physical changes in the bathroom might include grip bars properly installed on the wall, a hand-held spray unit, and a bath seat. These things aren't particularly expensive, but they do make a difference for someone who no longer can stand up while showering.

A raised seat on the toilet makes it easier to sit down and get up for someone whose leg strength is compromised. This can mean the difference between your loved one feeling utterly helpless and functioning more normally.

Everyone has a different view of what constitutes comfort. We learn what that view is by asking our loved ones what they want to do. And we don't ask just once. As circumstances change, we continue to ask our loved ones what they want us to do for them.

CHAPTER SIX -- I WASN'T PREPARED FOR THIS GIG

Every rock star band manager starts out as an amateur and becomes a professional through experience, often earning credits at the School of Hard Knocks. The person responsible for looking out for the band's best interests is very often someone who falls into the role over time and learns by trial and error.

If you don't have great managerial skills yet as a caregiver and you're unfamiliar with how the health care business works, you might feel overwhelmed by your responsibilities. It's hard to know exactly what you're supposed to do for your loved one and how you're supposed to do it.

Rock star caregivers might make the job seem easy, but that is rarely the case. Most of us direct ourselves to be stalwart and stout-hearted throughout our loved one's ordeal, but that doesn't mean our knees don't knock when we come across new situations that flummox us.

What we do well is we focus on the tools of companionship, compassion, comfort, and care because we understand that being seriously ill is a very scary thing. We work hard to make sure the patient has as much quality of life as is possible under the circumstances.

If you wonder whether it matters if the patient is satisfied with the care situation, ask yourself this question. What would *you* want from people who love you if you were seriously ill? How would you feel if you didn't get it?

Many people jump into caregiving without actually considering just how involved the process is. In effect, you are the "go-to" person for someone whose life has taken a bad turn, someone who is incredibly vulnerable physically, emotionally, and even mentally.

When people are stressed and distressed by the ravages of illness, it takes its toll on the whole person. Feeling weak or fragile is devastating to your psyche. All those wonderful things you could do before illness struck are suddenly gone. You live every day with uncertainty. Will you get better? Will you get worse? Will you wind up alone, because healthy people abandon you when you can't keep up?

Do you see now why being a rock star caregiver can mean the difference between *real* support and comfort for your loved one and "generic care"? If you leave it to other people take care of your seriously ill loved one, they don't necessarily have a vested interest in the outcome the way you do. Physical, emotional, and mental capabilities often fluctuate during illness. People who don't know your loved one might not catch the evolving deterioration of your loved one's normally sunny personality or see the sharp increase in pain that is experienced. They might not recognize the loss of hope and faith, or detect the rising frustration and anger your loved one goes through as health declines. Those changes aren't always resolved with medicine. Having clear lines of communication and understanding your loved one's perspective will help you to find practical solutions to enhance quality of life.

That's not to say that you can't or shouldn't hire people to help you provide care. Certainly band managers hire support staff to get the performers onto the stage or into the recording studio. It's normally a win-win. Caregivers often need help to physically care for a loved one with a serious illness. Finding the right balance is what a good manager does. You aren't managing your loved one or your loved one's disease. You're managing the various medical and support services that your loved one needs to have quality of life.

But to completely turn over the reins to someone who doesn't understand your loved one as a person the way you do...is that what you really want to do? You, as the main caregiver, are invested in making sure your loved one *feels the love*. You have a history with this person, a bond. You're in it together, come rain or come shine. Sure, other people can take care of the physical issues that crop up for someone who is seriously ill, but who will provide the love if it's not you? Love really is a healing ointment for someone who is hurting.

If you accept responsibility for making sure your loved one's emotional needs are met, you will feel more confident when you bring others in to help provide physical care. There's no need to feel like you are abandoning your loved one. You'll still be available to make sure everything is working right. You might also find that your loved one actually appreciates having other people help you with the physical caregiving.

How do you help a seriously patient to feel the love if you can't be there all the time? You do it by checking in regularly throughout the day and night. You make time to reach out and ascertain that things are going well. You do it by listening, by encouraging your loved one to be honest. You can't fix problems if you don't know they exist, can you? But above all else, you do it by being a good companion. Everybody needs a break from being sick. It's important to have fun, to connect apart from the dreary hours of illness. Those sweet moments will go a long way towards making your loved one feel better.

CHAPTER SEVEN -- WHAT HAPPENS OFFSTAGE

Rock stars sometimes become a commodity. A successful band is a money-making machine for the music company. Business people see dollar signs. The media scrum sees potential news stories in every snippet of gossip. The fans fantasize, imagining the glamorous lives their favorite rock stars lead. The bigger the success, the bigger the depersonalization of the individual as the public image grows. People stop caring about rock stars as human beings and begin to treat them like they are super beings. Think of Prince, Michael Jackson, and so many other music legends, whose lives were sadly lost because they were surrounded by managers and employees who were willing to enable and encourage dangerous behaviors in exchange for the chance to hang out in their celestial orbit and share the wealth. Rock stars need real love and honest people to help them stay grounded.

THE PRACTICAL CAREGIVER'S GUIDE TO ROCK STAR CAREGIVING

Like rock legends, ordinary people can sometimes become a commodity in the world of medicine, especially when they are seriously ill. Some doctors have trouble seeing beyond the test results, the blood counts, and the disease staging. Instead of focusing on quality of life for each patient, some doctors push for treatments that produce revenue, but leave their patients more vulnerable as a result. For many heart patients, having an implantable cardioverter defibrillator implanted is life-saving. But for a frail patient with serious heart failure, it can be painful and frightening to have the device shock the heart when it begins to fail. That's one reason why it's really important for your loved one to understand how new treatments are going to impact his or her life. What are the up sides and down sides of the procedures?

That's why it's so important that rock star caregivers understand the role they play in the lives of seriously ill patients. Sometimes the choices our loved ones face are less than ideal. Having a trusted confidant to share information with and to get feedback from can make a huge difference in outcome. You may not always have the answers, but by listening and understanding what your loved one wants to do, you open the door to a better quality of life.

That's the power of real love for seriously ill patients. We have a vested interest in making sure they get what they need. When they hurt, we hurt. When they feel better, we feel better. We are willing to put our own lives on "pause" until we know they're going to be okay.

Unfortunately, a cure is not possible with some diseases and illnesses. A disease can slowly progress over years or, sadly, go haywire in just weeks and months. It's not always easy to predict what will happen next. But we must never lose sight of the fact that while there is life, there is a human being in need of dignity and respect.

You probably already recognize your own sacrifices as a caregiver. But as hard as you work at taking care of your loved one, he or she is always working that much harder just to survive. That's the nature of the beast we call illness. Your rock star patient has to find a way to get through every grueling day. How do human beings motivate themselves to go through that daily grind of pain, frustration, and heartache of being seriously ill? When breathing, walking, and sleeping cease to come naturally to our loved ones, everything is harder.

Your acts of kindness, your tender mercies, and your inner strength play a huge role in helping your loved one get through the hardships. Your presence is reassuring when life is so uncertain. You toll behind the scenes to smooth catastrophes over, to soothe jagged nerves, to make sure things get done properly, so that your loved one has what is needed physically, emotionally, and mentally to get through the difficult days and nights. People might never know what you've been through, but you'll know. You'll carry it with you into the future. You will come to appreciate that you make a difference in the life of your loved one. When there is sorrow, dry the tears. Where there is anger, withstand the storm. Bring joy and laughter into the darkness and there is life again.

CHAPTER EIGHT -- LIFE IN A FISH BOWL

When you become a rock star caregiver, it's a given that you're no longer top banana. It's not that you don't matter, because you do. This is about priorities and whose needs carry greater weight. Your role as a caregiver is critical, even as you stand a little bit behind your loved one on the stage.

Think of it this way. Someone always takes the lead in every good band. Hootie rocked it on stage, but he would have been nothing without the Blowfish. Freddie Mercury made Queen famous with his songs, his stage persona, and his voice, but he relied heavily on his fellow musicians to create the group's unique sound. Steven Tyler has always been the face of Aerosmith...literally...but it wasn't called the Steve Tyler Band.

There is one important difference between rock stars and people who need caregivers. People choose to be performers, but nobody chooses to be seriously ill. That's the twist of fate that changes everything and everyone. Illness is what it is. For many people who are facing serious health threats, the "show must go on" philosophy can be a coping strategy that works to maintain self-respect, self-achievement, self-esteem, and a continued sense of purpose. It also helps to ground a seriously ill person in reality. We begin to understand that we are on this earth only for a short time and we must work quickly to achieve our dreams.

Think of the pressure that rock stars face when they're on tour. Hot or cold, sick or well, they are expected to show up for every concert date in every city where they are scheduled to perform. They have to put on a happy face and belt out those tunes, whether they feel like something the cat dragged in or they feel like they're on top of the world. People bought tickets to see them and they want their money's worth. It costs a lot of money to produce a concert. There is a lot of preparation work involved, from marketing to security. The outlay of money before a rock star ever takes to the stage is significant. Nobody wants to give refunds to ticket buyers or to reschedule the show unless it's absolutely necessary.

Rock stars find themselves abandoned when fickle fans turn their attention to the next rock sensation. One day, people can't get enough of you and your music. Your songs go platinum. You're on the cover of *Rolling Stone* and you're hitting all the late night shows to do interviews. And then, you fall out of the sky like a meteorite, smacking into the hard, unyielding ground. What changed? What did you do wrong?

The music business exists solely to fulfill the public's demand to be entertained. In order to tour and to record as musicians, the band has to have fans. But fan adoration is not the same thing as *real* love. It's often based on shallow emotions, superficial perceptions, and skin-deep judgments. We connect to particular songs because they reflect something we're going through at that moment in time. We like those wild riffs on guitar and the drum solos that our favorite performers play because they sound and look "cool". Whatever attracts us to our favorite rock stars isn't a true human-to-human experience. We may like and respect their work, but they don't really know us and we don't really know them.

Patients sometimes have a similar experience when the public finds out they are struggling to survive. There can be a tremendous sense of social pressure and sometimes even a stigma attached to being in poor health. People find themselves struggling to keep their jobs as their disease progresses. Sometimes, after many sick days and a physical inability to carry out one's duties, it's necessary to step down.

But it can always get worse. Believe it or not, some folks will abandon a person who is seriously ill. Those insensitive clouts will say, "I can't be around sick people," as they flee to the hills. A few might even have a twinge or two of guilt when they utter those words. The hurt often goes deep when this happens.

But in reality, it's not really about your loved one at all. These fair-weather folks are desperate to escape the dark cloud of mortality they perceive in that moment in time. The fact is we're all going to die at some point. Our time on Earth is limited. But where there is life, we should embrace every precious moment and enjoy it to the fullest. Why waste it on shallow people who really don't know, understand, or appreciate what your loved one has gone through and will continue to go through?

But as a society, some well-meaning actions can create stress for our loved ones. Cheering for someone who is ill can feel good when you're on the outside looking in. But if you are the patient, the pressure you might feel when people express their confidence that you are or will be cured can be hard to bear. You can feel like a failure. You can feel wounded by the deep disappointment. Yes, some people do recover. But serious illness is what it is. Not all patients bounce back from such a life-changing event. Rarely does anyone ever get through it unscathed. A patient can follow every doctor's order, take every medication prescribed, go through every treatment, but still not recover. This is *never* a patient's fault.

This is all the more reason to surround your loved one with confident, compassionate people who understand that we shouldn't worry about whether our loved one will be cured. We should focus on the here-and-now, because that's all we know for certain that we have. Work at making every moment that comes along a good one and embrace the opportunities to live life out loud. Life is short, so it's up to us to make it sweet.

CHAPTER NINE -- GROUPIES, SICKIES, AND NEEDIES

Rock stars have groupies, those super-fans who like to follow the band from club to club and concert to concert. They hang out at the hotels where the rock stars are staying, in the hopes of having the opportunity to party with the band. Do they really have real personal relationships with the groups? No. If they did, they wouldn't be groupies. They would be friends. The relationships between them would be mutual and equal. But groupies aren't looking for real relationships. They're into fantasies with benefits.

Just like rock stars have groupies, sometimes seriously ill patients have sickies who seek them out. The sickies will drive you crazy with all of their supposed knowledge about illness. They'll call just before your loved one has surgery to discuss what happened to So-and-So when *she* had that procedure (it's always a horror story). They'll inform you just how bad your loved one's prognosis is because they read all about it on the Internet. Do yourself a favor. Say, "Hold that thought a minute!" and run as far and as fast from the sickies as you can. No seriously ill patient ever needs to consult with a sickie about health care matters, and I dare say healthy people are wise to avoid them as well.

One thing is true about sickies. They're never interested in what your loved one *needs* or what your loved one *feels*. They're likely to burnish their social status by sharing your personal information with the public. They embellish the limited facts they have access to in order to add drama effect to their stories. "Have you heard about Whazz-Her-Name? I was just talking to her family the other day. She's only got less than three months to live!"

Like the overzealous sickies who get a thrill from knowing someone who is seriously ill, there are the super-needies that show up at the most inopportune times. They're the "Chicken Littles" of the disease world, seeking your attention with their "Oh woe is me!" plaintive. They are incapable of empathy or compassion for your loved one's plight. They want you and your loved one to reassure *them*, to make *them* feel better about your loved one's illness. They can't wrap their heads around what's happening because *they're* worried sick. When is your loved one going to die? Do you know when will the funeral be? Escape their nets of neediness. It's not your job to help *them* deal with their emotions about your loved one's serious illness. You already have a job, and that's to take care of your loved one. You don't need this kind of distraction.

What you and your loved one *do* need, however, is a solid support circle. Fill it with those people who genuinely care and are ready to help. Don't feel guilty that you need them. When they offer it to you, accept it with a grateful heart and welcome them in. These are the people who will lift you up and help you to keep going when you are at rock bottom.

CHAPTER TEN -- IT'S NOT ALL ABOUT YOU AND YET IT IS

Not all rock stars handle fame and fortune well. For some, the minute they start to get notice for their music, it all starts to spiral out of control. There are "incidents" and "episodes" involving wild behavior and illegal activities. We're always shocked to learn that there's been a tragic car accident, or an unexpected death due to an overdose. Life in the fast lane is...well, it's fast.

The spotlight seems to draw some rock stars like moths to the flame. They become so greedy, so determined to be the center of attention, they forget that other people even exist. They are always the most important people in any room, at least in their own minds. Their entourages feed this belief by meekly following them about and acquiescing to every demand they put forth, even the ones that are outrageous and ridiculous.

Having people fawn all over you, willing to do your bidding, is a heady experience. You start to believe that you deserve all that special attention. Surrounded by "go-fers", who indulge your every whim, your ego grows by leaps and bounds. When egos and tempers collide with reality, it can spell disaster. The unbalanced and unequal relationship is so skewed that people lose sight of what the human heart needs. The rock star controls the universe and everyone orbits around him or her.

When people are seriously ill, their needs are often so great that caregivers tend to lose themselves in the care they provide. It's easy to forget who *you* are when your loved one has emergency after emergency. Slowly but surely, you seem to fade away as a person.

While you are caring for your rock star patient, you need to feed your own goals, your own hopes, and your own dreams. You have to keep true to who *you* are as a human being, and that means stepping away for some *me* time every day.

Is it really necessary? Yes. Caregiving can drain you of every ounce of energy you have. Your loved one is dependent upon you for the care you provide. What happens if you become overwhelmed and you can't cope anymore? Many caregivers have run out of steam because they forgot to take care of themselves and their own needs. Post traumatic stress is a very real threat to those who don't take the time to process their own thoughts, emotions, and frustrations in real time. You have to have a clear head and a clear heart to be an effective caregiver.

You might not even recognize the danger signs along the road because you're so distracted by the challenges of your loved one's illness now. Back when you and your loved one were both healthy, the flow of energy went back and forth between you. There was give-and-take. You engaged in activities that were reciprocal.

But caregiving requires you to subjugate yourself to your loved one's need for care. There are many times when your own (very real) needs are less important than those of your loved one. By necessity, your loved one takes...and takes...and takes, while you give...and give...and give. It's not that your loved one doesn't *want* to give to you. It's that your loved one's illness steals so much precious time and energy, there's often little left over to give to you.

Where, then, do you get the nurturing that you need, if your loved one can no longer provide it? You have to give it back to yourself by taking daily breaks that recharge your batteries.

Separating yourself from your caregiving during break time allows you to de-stress. If you take an hour to go to the gym or to take a hike, you can get physical exercise *and* clear your head. That will enable you to return with a better attitude and help you maintain your own health.

If you think you can't squeeze a break in because things are so tenuous for your loved one, there's no need to leave home. Give yourself fifteen minutes here, fifteen minutes there, to de-pressurize. Step into another room to read a magazine, catch up on emails, or call a friend. Take a long, hot shower or bath and pamper yourself. Prune some tree branches or putter in the garden. Toss a ball to the dog or shoot some baskets in your driveway. Better still, find a peaceful spot to sit and read that book that's been sitting on your "to read" shelf all these months. You use the time to engage in something *you* enjoy doing. That *me* time is yours and yours alone.

CHAPTER ELEVEN -- CAN YOU DIE FROM STAGE FRIGHT?

Performing live for large audiences can be nerve-racking for rock stars. The public tends to think that singers take to the stage and enjoy the whole concert process from start to finish. That's not necessarily so. Adele has talked openly about her struggle to overcome performance jitters. Her biggest fear is that she will let her fans down. She's so affected by stage fright that she's no longer sure she'll ever be able to tour again.

Rod Stewart, Justin Bieber, and Rihanna have had their own moments of panic. They are just a few of the performers known to suffer from that paralyzing fear one gets from performing for crowds.

Part of the pressure comes from the public. When people put you up on a pedestal and expect you to perform every note flawlessly, it can be tough to measure up every day.

But there is also the internal pressure that the singers put upon themselves. Their anxious thoughts start to crowd their heads with so much "noise" that they just can't focus.

If the audiences are large, there's a greater chance that a performer will panic as he or she stares out at the sea of unrecognizable faces. Nobody wants to be booed off the stage. Rejection can hurt.

The secret to overcoming stage fright is to make a human connection. When you focus on a few of the happy faces of people in the audience, you can see that people are enjoying what you are doing. You no longer notice the thousands of eyes staring at you, watching every move you make and judging you. Support is very important to performers.

Patients also need friendly faces and support to help them stay on course. Imagine using every ounce of your energy to hobble across a sidewalk on your way from the car to the entrance of a store. It's an exhausting process, so you have to take your time. You pause and look up in time to find an acquaintance staring at you, a shocked expression on her face. That's when you realize you're not the "old" you any more. Now your illness frightens people, leaving you to wonder: "Do I really look that awful?"

The difference between stage fright and the fear that accompanies a serious illness is that you can avoid stage fright by canceling the performance, but you can't avoid the fear that accompanies serious illness. It follows you wherever you go.

That fear affects people in different ways. There are so many variables that affect patient survival, including the side effects of the treatments, your physical condition, the complications that can knock you back, and even whether or not your immune system is strong enough to get through it all.

But a patient's personality also plays a role in dealing with that fear. Some patients withdraw emotionally, unable to cope. Some rage against their fate, furious that this is happening to them. Others pretend it's all some terrible mistake and they will wake up tomorrow to find everything is back to normal, but that version of tomorrow never comes and they are left to ponder how long they will be able to deny reality.

Fear is usually contagious, passing from person to person, until it is stopped in its tracks. Rock star caregivers learn to be perceptive and receptive, offering a shoulder to cry on, a hand to hold, and a calm demeanor. You might have your own worries about how things are going, but you're wise enough to not dump them onto your loved one's weak shoulders. When you are overwhelmed, you step out and get a handle on things. You seek your own wise counselor to help you cope. Learn what the options are for your loved one in terms of comfort, so that you can introduce them when your loved one is hurting.

CHAPTER TWELVE -- HOW DID WE FALL INTO THIS HOLE?

Some rock stars on the road follow Alice down the rabbit hole, into a world that makes no sense. Instead of sleeping at night, they go to bed as the sun comes up. Instead of working during the day, they're up all night. They can't sleep, so they take a pill for that. They have no energy, so they take another one to wake themselves up. As the tour continues, they become more disoriented with every twist in the road.

Living with a serious illness can also feel surreal, especially with all the medications you might take to manage your symptoms. Whether you're dealing with the fog of pain pills, the dizziness that comes with taking blood pressure and heart medications, or the neuropathy and confusion that comes with taking some chemotherapy drugs, you can wind up feeling like you're having bizarre out-of-body experiences. There's no way to know what might happen next. Over time, the constant stress of coping with that uncertainty often pushes patients off course. It's not bad enough that you can feel the frightening changes that are occurring within your body. You also have to worry about what you're going to do when things worsen. You waste precious hours trying to imagine what *that* will be like. This is a roller coaster ride through hell. Every the future creeps closer, like a dark cloud of doom.

Patients are sometimes so upset by the news that things aren't good, they don't absorb the information the doctors provide during medical appointments. Later on, they might recall the information incorrectly, thinking that they know what they were told. One way to overcome these miscommunications is to take notes about what the physician says, so you can walk your loved one back through it when he or she is mentally and emotionally ready. The best way to do this is to present the positive aspects of the appointment first. The human brain needs that message of hope to frame the changes.

As a rock star caregiver, it's also important for you to understand that your loved one is likely to pick up on your signals. Are you unintentionally transmitting your anxiety about the situation? Sorting out your own emotions will help you to offer an even-handed view of the current changes.

Another pitfall for caregivers is to push a loved one to be a good sport, to "cheer up" about being in poor health. Very often patients feel frustrated, disappointed, and even angry at their own bodies succumbing to illness. If the body isn't functioning well, everything is a struggle. It's hard to have a positive attitude under those conditions. Coming to grips with having a serious illness is an ongoing physical, emotional, and mental process. It takes effort to find balance and stability with the "new normal". That doesn't happen right away. Patients need to make peace with their health in their own time, in their own way.

While it may be tempting to avoid starting any conversation that involves talking about negative feelings and unpleasant experiences, it's important to give your loved one the chance to speak openly and honestly about what's going on. Knowing you are there to listen can be reassuring and comforting. You don't have to have all the answers. It's not your job to fix this. But by listening to your loved one, you might just learn something that helps you figure out better ways to provide comfort. Distressing physical symptoms tend to trigger panic in seriously ill patients. They sometimes perceive these changes to be indicative of a worsening of their situation. Feeling physically better usually reduces the accompanying mental and emotional anguish, enabling patients to cope more effectively with the status quo. That's why it's important to focus your efforts on finding comfort for your loved one.

CHAPTER THIRTEEN -- I USED TO BE SOMEBODY

When rock star legends are starting out, they have a vision of themselves as successes. They imagine themselves up there on the stage, playing their songs for the adoring masses. They see themselves in the recording studio, cranking out the tunes. It's not hard for them to picture their names on the Billboard charts for hit after hit after hit. But what happens when their popularity plummets and the stardust burns up as it falls through the stratosphere? After the ticket sales drop, and the recording contracts end, some musicians fall off the cliff of fame and fortune, winding up in the dark abyss of despair and desperation.

Real life is scary when your charmed life ends and your nightmares begin. Even rock legends will feel that pain because they are human beings. They need good people around them to help them switch gears when they reinvent themselves and rise once more.

Some former rock stars have become music producers, promoting new talent. Some have become composers, scoring music for movies or television. Some change careers completely. Who would have predicted that Daryl Hall, of Hall and Oates fame, would become an antique house renovator, receiving as much respect and accolades for his building skills as for his music? Or that Terry Chimes of The Clash would become a chiropractor because he enjoys helping people heal? Jeff "Skunk" Baxter, of Doobie Brothers and Steely Dan fame, has not only continued to work in the music business, he started a successful second career as a systems analyst and consultant for US missile defense (I'll bet you never saw that one coming!) And how did Brian May, the lead guitarist for Queen fare? It only took him forty years to become an astrophysicist. He started his Ph.D. in 1971 and finally finished it in 2007.

Sometimes it takes a while for seriously ill people to come to terms with their "new normal" because it requires some reinventing of self and life. Some patients might not be able to drive anymore. That can have a big impact on activities they engage in. Some patients have to scale back their careers, switching to part-time work or working from home at least some of the time. Others find that they can't continue their employment and have to retire, which can be a bitter pill to swallow until your loved one figures out how to make this new life work.

While your loved one is adjusting to "the new normal", you will have to do some adjusting of your own. At some point, you, too, will have to rethink how to manage your own activities, especially at those times when your loved one's need for care increases and uses up more of your time. It helps to be flexible and creative in your approach.

Some caregivers believe that, in order to be effective, they have to become subordinate to their loved ones. They surrender who and what they are in favor of devoting themselves unselfishly to patients who need care. You and your loved one had a relationship before illness interfered. No doubt the inter-play between you was dynamic and interesting. Don't give that up. The biggest mistake a caregiver can make is to let life come to a screeching halt.

Maybe you feel guilty that your loved one can't participate, or your loved one feels that it's unfair that you get to go off and do things separately. Maybe you think that you *must* spend all your time with him or her, lest you be viewed as a rat (who among us hasn't cringed when hearing those dreaded words, "You're leaving me?"). Lose that guilt by recognizing that you're not being selfish in looking after yourself. You're actually helping yourself to re-energize. You will keep your brain sharper, so you can quickly gather your wits about you in a crisis. It will actually make you a better caregiver.

CHAPTER FOURTEEN -- CELEBRITY SIGHTINGS AND OTHER FREAK OUTS

For rock stars, fame and fortune might be the perks of a successful rock career, but there are also dues to pay. When you're a public figure, you have little expectation of privacy. Life can quickly become strange when people stop treating you like a human being and start treating you like you're the Last Jedi in the galaxy. All eyes stare at you whenever you walk down the street. People watch your every move expectantly. What's it like to face such constant scrutiny? It's unnerving. Do you run home and bolt the door to keep the world out? Brian Wilson, of Beach Boys fame, is a recluse who doesn't want to be bothered. John "Cougar" Mellencamp wrestled with agoraphobia that kept him cooped up at home. Carly Simon, Barbra Streisand, and Naomi Judd have all experienced panic attacks over the years that kept them from venturing out in public.

For people who are dealing with a serious illness, this need to escape public scrutiny can be very real too. Cancer sometimes attacks your body with frightening ferocity, and the change in your appearance can be a cruel reminder that you're all too mortal. Whether there are radiation or chemo side effects, surgical scars, or a combination of these, there is no escaping the evidence that your body was assaulted by the disease. Every time you pass by a mirror, you remember. So does everyone else.

But a disease like cancer can be even crueler to your psyche. Its abuse knows no bounds. It hovers at your shoulder. It reminds you that you don't know how much time you have left. Is it months or years? Will there be a cure in time or will you become an annual statistic cited in a newspaper report? Sometimes you just need to put some distance between you and the disease. Where can you go to escape it?

If you're a patient, you might think that you will feel better when you go out for breakfast at your favorite hangout. But imagine walking in to find that everyone is staring at you because you're wearing a chemo cap on your head or leaning on a cane. They notice that your clothes are too big because you lost so much weight. It's not your imagination that those eyes are watching you or that people are whispering behind your back.

As a rock star caregiver, you need to understand the situation from a human perspective. Just as they would gossip about a celebrity's shocking face lift or a politician's sudden fifty-pound weight gain, friends and acquaintances react to physical changes they see in people they know by trying to figure out what caused the change. They often speculate. Is there a divorce in the works? Did she suffer a nervous breakdown after her only child left for college? Did that guy really lose all of his money after his investments tanked? Most of the time, people are clueless, but that doesn't stop them from trying to get to the bottom of the mystery.

If it's a good change, there's usually a celebratory cheer. But when it's a bad change and they are caught off-guard, people sometimes are less than sensitive. Some, in fact, say the most idiotic and absurd things to seriously ill patients.

For that reason, it's important for you to be aware of what might happen, so that you can steer your loved one away from potentially uncomfortable situations. Be mindful of your loved one's emotional stamina when you go out in public. Nobody enjoys a helping of pity served with an order of pancakes. That kind of attention is unwelcome, whether you're a rock star or a person with a serious illness.

We human beings seek peace of mind in times of crisis; we need a little distance between us and the constant reminder of illness. We need to forget about things we cannot control long enough to remember what life without it felt like, because we are working to get back there. The trouble is it's hard to do when the disease comes with us wherever we go. To see the fear, anxiety, and worry reflected in the eyes of people who know us is tough to take. Nobody ever "allows" a disease to invade the body (as if this is ever a choice). It's the luck of the draw. It really could happen to anybody, even you and me.

That negative public perception of your loved one's situation will affect how he or she feels about it. It's hard to stay hopeful when people take a look at you and assume that you're on death's doorstep. When they suddenly change the way they treat you, that's a hurt that goes deep. This is why many seriously ill patients avoid their old haunts in favor of eateries where they won't run into people they know. Can you really blame them?

Rock star caregivers understand the pain this can cause our loved ones. We work hard to provide them with opportunities to enjoy activities that make them *feel good* about life. If you think your loved one can't handle the bad reactions that take place in public spaces, why put him or her in the position of enduring them? Take the bull by the horns and be a positive influencer. Suggest a new adventure to a different greasy spoon or pancake house. "I've got a hankering to try something new. What about you? I heard about this little place across the river...."

CHAPTER FIFTEEN -- CHAMPIONING A CAUSE ONLY WORKS IF IT FIXES A PROBLEM

You might think it's bad advice to avoid people you know. Maybe you have that "hero" gene and you feel the need to set people straight. If you're tempted to wait until someone gets out of line with your loved one, planning an ambush of the bad behavior, consider how it will affect your loved one. Sure, you may feel noble telling off some twit who babbles about how awful your loved one looks. You might even give in to the urge to shout angrily at the retreating back of someone who couldn't bear to look at your loved one when you passed in the grocery store. But is that how you change what is wrong? By the time you're done laying out the miscreant in lavender, your loved one's emotional turmoil will be increased ten fold.

Truth be told, you are trying to swim upstream with someone who doesn't have the energy to make the journey. Your loved one is *very* ill. Is this really the time and place to confront public foibles? Will you really change the world by correcting someone's sad social faux pas? Sometimes the path of least resistance is the kinder, gentler choice.

If you really care about providing good support to your loved one in public, go proactive in productive ways. Why not invite a compassionate friend...or two...or three to join you? Engage in activities with people you trust to lift your loved one's spirits. Grab a corner table at a relaxing cafe and spend an hour talking over fun times. Go to a movie matinee, when the theater isn't crowded, and see a light-hearted movie together. Visit a museum, an aquarium, or a nature center as a group and share the excitement of discovering something new. Pack a picnic and take a drive to the beach, the mountains, or the river. Be social, but do it wisely, with a purpose in mind. When you and your loved one go out in the world in a safe way, you're helping your loved one to stay connected to life.

There's a real benefit to expanding your territory beyond your usual neighborhood. It's common for strangers to avoid making eye contact. If you're among strangers, your loved one has fewer expectations of rejection. You don't have to pretend or to plaster a phony smile on your face. You can just be yourself.

But don't be surprised if you come occasionally across some friendly people along the way. They're the ones who have walked in your shoes, or those of your loved one. They understand the frustrations and upsets along the road. They also understand that a smile and some cheerful banter can light up the heart.

Does it sound like this kind of management style will turn you into a control freak, as you try to stave off any unpleasant and unnecessary incidents that could affect your loved one's mood? Congratulations, rock star caregiver, for recognizing a very important function of your job. It's okay to shoo away the unnecessary stress in favor of providing comfort and kindness. "Cocooning" is a pleasant way of controlling the environment your loved one is subjected to, and yes, it's very much a form of protection. You are, in effect, wrapping your loved one in a cozy experience that will send a very strong message to the heart and mind: "I still see you as a person who need to have fun, even with all your challenges. Let's do this."

By eliminating the potentially negative emotional reminders of your loved one's illness out in public, you're actually helping to improve his or her outlook. Isn't that what a good rock band manager does when he or she puts some distance between the overly intrusive fans and the stressed-out rock star, or intervenes between the nosy Parkers in the press and the exhausted rock star? Life on the road can be grueling. A good band manager tries to eliminate the unwelcome distractions, so that the rock star can unwind and relax off-stage.

Look back on all the medical interventions, appointments, and treatments your loved one has been subjected to in the last year. Every time you two set foot in a hospital, cancer center, or physician's office, it was for a procedure of some kind, wasn't it? Your loved one goes through all that rigmarole for the chance to survive this challenging illness. But that's only a small part of what your loved one needs to heal.

Consider, too, how many patients you and your loved one have seen in medical settings. If the only people you came in contact with were patients and doctors, how does that impact your loved one's psyche? Being surrounded by people that are seriously ill, especially when some of them lose their battles, hardly inspires your loved one to stay hopeful.

It's important to be out in the real world, where you are not constantly surrounded by reminders of what illness does to people. Sure, the body may have taken a big hit, but your loved one is more than just a body. Your loved one needs to feel like a whole person.

Deliberately controlling the environment around your loved one can help to reduce stress and anxiety. People who are seriously ill spend so much time trying to just survive that they don't have any spare energy to fend off any unnecessary negativity. What energy they do have should be reinforced by positive experiences that bolster a better attitude and hope for the future. Those good feelings go a long way towards improving the quality of life that is so critical for seriously ill people to enjoy. Getting out and about gives both of you the chance to bond in positive ways and to talk about something other than what medication is causing unpleasant side effects and what the next round of chemotherapy is going to be like.

CHAPTER SIXTEEN -- WHAT A LONG, STRANGE TRIP IT'S BEEN

There is no escaping the fact that illness has altered life as you both know it. You have come a long way as a team and forged new bonds as human beings. When you can look back on your time as a caregiver and see positive experiences mingled among the terrifying or the painful moments, you will know that you helped to provide quality of life.

And if, in reflection, you can recognize personal growth in both yourself and your loved one, that's further evidence that disease did not steal everything from the two of you. You held your own and you found ways to rise above.

Think about the rock songs that resonate with us years after their releases. The melodies and lyrics make us *feel* something genuine. They give us back our sense of wonder about love and life. Or they tap into our hope that things will work out, even as the dark clouds gather. We are moved to connect to one another in good ways. Or we abandon our old lives because we understand they didn't work for us.

How many of us hear that old Gloria Gaynor song, *I Will Survive* (written by Freddie Perren and Dino Fekaris) and feel empowered? The song first came out in 1978 and tapped a nerve in so many people. That's because it's about surviving something horrible and coming out on top. "At first I was afraid, I was petrified...."

Or we hear Chaka Khan singing the 1984 hit, *Through the Fire*, (David Foster, Tom Keane, Cynthia Weil) and we understand what it's like to come out of an experience that has challenged us to find the strength we never knew we had. "Through the fire, to the limit, to the wall...." We took the risk, just for the chance to be with someone who mattered to us. We made it because we set our sights on being resilient...brave...strong.

And how can we not be inspired by the 1987 Aretha Franklin and George Michael rendition of *I Knew You Were Waiting* (Simon Climie and Dennis Morgan)? "Like a warrior that fights, and wins the battle, I know the taste of victory...." Anyone who has gone through night consumed by shadows understands how scary life can be.

As human beings, we have to believe that we can conquer these terrible times in our lives. We have to believe that our spirits are greater than the challenges we face. If we don't, we can't fight back or rise above. We are defeated before we start and doomed, like lemmings, to jump off the edge of the cliff and disappear forever. We won't even stand up and face the horizon. How can there be quality of life where there is no hope, no joy, and no love to get us through the darkness?

Believing that we can get through these hardships is half the battle. If we think we can, we will try to find a way. William Shakespeare's character, Lady Macbeth, says in *Macbeth*: "But screw your courage to the sticking-place, and we'll not fail." Sometimes when we are dealing with all the wild twists and turns that serious illness can bring to our lives, courage is all we have left. If we are willing to seek better days for our loved ones as they battle on, and if we set our sights on the quality of life for our loved ones, on the laughter and love we keep in our hearts, the journey we take together will be memorable. Life is, after all, what we make of it. Let there be music.

ABOUT THE AUTHOR

Sara M. Barton, who trained as an educator, interacted with hospitalized children during her first teaching practicum in the pediatric department of a large city hospital, gaining insight into the value of play therapy and socialization during medical treatment. With minors in art and psychology, she later worked with adult patients in a psychiatric admissions hospital and disturbed adolescents in residential care. These experiences were invaluable when caring for her mother over more than a decade. She created the Practical Caregiver Guides website and Practical Caregiver blogs to help family caregivers:

Practical Caregiver Guides Website for Family Caregivers:

https://practicalcaregiverguides.org

Sara M. Barton is the author of several fast-paced cozy mysteries featuring lively characters: *The Scarlet Wilson Mysteries, The Off the Books Mysteries, The International Killer Chefs Competition Mysteries* (The first book in the new series is entitled *Frosted!*)You can find her author website at: https://smbarton.com

\

www.ingramcontent.com/pod-product-compliance
Lightning Source LLC
Chambersburg PA
CBHW030047230526
45471CB00003B/978